C000070045

My Mediterranean Meals & Veggies Cooking Guide

Creative and Healthy
Mediterranean Recipes

Mateo Buscema

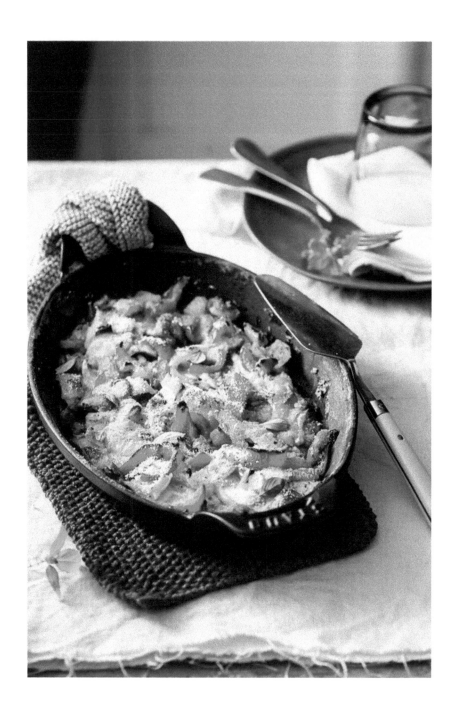

© Copyright 2021 - All rights reserved.

The content contained within this book may not be reproduced, duplicated or transmitted without direct written permission from the author or the publisher.
Under no circumstances will any blame or legal responsibility be held against the publisher, or author, for any damages, reparation, or monetary loss due to the information contained within this book. Either directly or indirectly.

Legal Notice:
This book is copyright protected. This book is only for personal use. You cannot amend, distribute, sell, use, quote or paraphrase any part, or the content within this book, without the consent of the author or publisher.

Disclaimer Notice:
Please note the information contained within this document is for educational and entertainment purposes only. All effort has been executed to present accurate, up to date, and reliable, complete information. No warranties of any kind are declared or implied. Readers acknowledge that the author is not engaging in the rendering of legal, financial, medical or professional advice. The content within this book has been derived from various sources. Please consult a licensed professional before attempting any techniques outlined in this book.
By reading this document, the reader agrees that under no circumstances is the author responsible for any losses, direct or indirect, which are incurred as a result of the use of information contained within this document, including, but not limited to, — errors, omissions, or inaccuracies.

TABLE OF CONTENTS

Fluffy carrot broccoli fritters

Ingredients

- ¼ cup of Panko Breadcrumbs
- 1.1 lb. of Broccoli Head
- 4 Carrots
- Sunflower Oil
- ¼ teaspoon of Black Pepper
- 4 tablespoons of Plain Flour
- 1 cup of Flat Leaf Parsley
- 3 Eggs, Separated
- 1 teaspoon of Pink Himalayan Salt

Directions

1. Chop broccoli in a roughly manner and process in a food processor.
2. In a bowl, combine the processed broccoli, carrots, breadcrumbs, salt, flour, black pepper, and egg yolks.
3. Beat the egg whites until firm.
4. Fold in the whites into the broccoli mixture.
5. Fry each fritter 3 minutes max on every side.
6. Keep adding bit of oil as you fry and or accordingly.
7. Serve with any dip and enjoy.

Spinach crepes with pan roasted vegetables

This recipe is entirely vegetarian with varieties of vegetables from spinach to mushrooms then to tomatoes making a flavorful lunch, dinner and or breakfast.

Ingredients

- 4 cups of fresh spinach
- 1 large egg
- 1 thumb-size piece of fresh ginger, grated
- 3 tablespoons of butter
- 1 medium onion
- 1 cup of milk
- 1 tablespoon of dried oregano
- 1 cup of grated cheese of your choice
- 2 cups of cherry tomatoes
- 1 teaspoon pink salt
- 1 cup of plain flour
- ½ teaspoon of pink salt
- Sunflower oil for frying
- 2 cups of chopped mushrooms
- 1 cup of grated cheese of your choice

- 1 yellow bell pepper
- 2 cups of chopped flat leaf parsley
- 3 garlic cloves

Directions

1. In a food processor, process the spinach together with the milk until smooth.
2. Transfer this to a mixing bowl.
3. Add together flour with salt, egg, and grated ginger. Mix to combine.
4. Next, heat your frying pan.
5. Then, add bit of oil.
6. Place in the batter
7. Spread evenly throughout the pan by turning around the pan.
8. Cook for 2 minutes on each sides

Pan-roasted vegetables

Ingredients

- Butter
- Onions
- Mushrooms
- Pepper
- Garlic
- Cherry tomatoes
- Parsley
- Grated cheese

Directions

1. Start by melting butter.
2. Add sliced onion, mushrooms and pepper into the pan.
3. Roast for 10 minutes then add the garlic with the cherry tomatoes.
4. Continue to roast for 3 minutes.
5. Turn off the heat then stir in parsley.
6. Next, fill the pancakes with vegetable mixture.
7. Sprinkle with grated cheese.
8. Serve and enjoy when warm.

Rice paper sushi

This recipe combines smoked salmon with variety of vegies.

Ingredients

- 1 cup of sushi rice
- 1/8 cup of rice vinegar
- ½ tablespoon of granulated sugar
- ½ teaspoon of salt
- 1 large ripe avocado
- 3 ounces of smoked salmon
- ½ cucumber
- 1 large carrot, peeled
- 4 rice paper wrappers

Directions

1. Begin by cooking the rice as per the package Directions.
2. In a mixing bowl, combine rice vinegar, sugar, and salt.
3. Stir to dissolve the sugar completely.
4. Pour over cooked rice and mix.
5. Let the rice cool.

6. As the rice cooks and cools, cut smoked salmon and avocado into strips whereas cut cucumber and carrot into thin matchsticks.
7. In a large skillet add warm water to submerge a rice paper wrapper until completely soft.
8. Take it out and put onto a clean worktop.
9. The rice paper should be covered with a layer of rice evenly except on the edges that should be left clear.
10. Place a layer of salmon, top this with half carrots, half cucumbers and avocado slices on the fillings.
11. Lift and place the rice paper over the fillings.
12. Roll over the fillings.
13. Slice the sushi sausage into bites.
14. Repeat this step for all the rice papers.

15. Serve and enjoy with soy sausage.

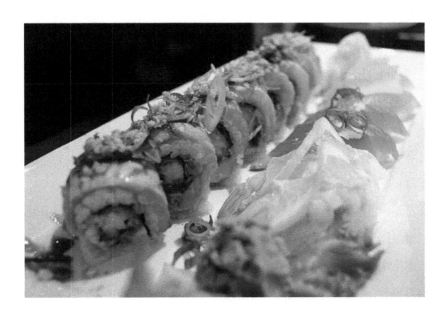

Pan fried asparagus with parmesan

This is a Mediterranean side dish, crunchy and tasty perfect for any kind of dinner.

Ingredients

- 2 tablespoons of ground almonds
- Salt and pepper
- 2 tablespoons of olive oil
- 9 ounces of asparagus spears
- 2 tablespoons of parmesan, grated

Directions

1. Heat up the oil in a skillet.
2. Place the spears into the pan touching the pan.
3. Season with a pinch of salt and black pepper.
4. Roast for 2 minutes each batch.
5. Turn every spear half of the time for even frying.
6. Transfer them onto a baking sheet.
7. Place together the grated Parmesan with ground almonds and sprinkle with the spears.
8. Shake to coat equally.
9. Taste and adjust accordingly.
10. Serve and enjoy immediately.

Butter roasted split pea power bowl

The butter roasted split pea power bowl is highly rated among quick tasty dishes and filling. It is rich in healthy fats, vitamins, and proteins.

Ingredients

- A handful of fresh flat leaf parsley
- 60g of feta cheese
- 1 cup of split peas
- 1 large ripe avocado
- 80g of smoked salmon
- Salt
- 30g of unsalted butter
- A squeeze of lemon

Directions

1. Firstly, begin by soaking your peas overnight in cold water.
2. Drain and shift them to a pot with 3 cups of water.
3. Boil for 15 minutes.

4. Lower the heat and let simmer for 20 minutes.

5. Drain any excess water.

6. Melt your butter over a medium heat.

7. Place in the drained peas.

8. Increase the heat, let it roast for 3 minutes, keep stirring occasionally.

9. Add roughly chopped parsley, let roast for 3 minutes.

10. Prepare the avocado.

11. Cut into slices.

12. Slice dice feta cheese.

13. Serve and enjoy.

Roasted fall vegetables

Ingredients

- 1 tablespoon of dried thyme
- 1 pound of cauliflower florets
- ¼ teaspoon of black pepper
- 1 teaspoon of salt
- ½ pound of carrots, sliced
- 1 pound of potatoes, cut into chunks
- 1 teaspoon of paprika
- ½ pound of sweet potatoes, cut into chunks
- 12 ounces of Brussels sprouts
- 1 teaspoon of garlic powder
- 1 onion, quartered
- 3 tablespoons of olive oil

Directions

1. Preheat your oven to 400°F.
2. Transfer cauliflower, potatoes, carrots, and Brussels sprouts into a large bowl.
3. Separate the onion layers. Leave 3 layers together.
4. Add to the bowl.
5. Then, drizzle the veggies with olive oil.
6. Sprinkle the seasoning and mix.

7. Shift veggies onto a large baking tray lined with baking parchment.
8. Bake at 400°F for 35 minutes, stirring occasionally.
9. Serve and enjoy.

Red cabbage coleslaw

Ingredients

- ¾ cup of mayonnaise
- 1 large carrot
- ½ teaspoon of salt
- 1 large celery stalk
- ¼ teaspoon of black pepper
- ½ small head red cabbage
- 1 tablespoon of vinegar
- 1 small onion, thinly sliced
- 2 tablespoons fresh lemon juice

Directions

1. In a large mixing bowl, combine every ingredient.
2. Mix thoroughly.
3. Let it chill
4. Serve and enjoy.

Parmentier potatoes

These are tasty cubed potatoes tossed with herbs and olive oil. They are roasted until crispy in an oven.

Ingredients

- black pepper
- 2 pounds of potatoes, peeled
- 2 teaspoon of dried rosemary
- 2 tablespoons of olive oil
- Salt
- 1 teaspoon of dried parsley

Directions

1. Preheat your oven to 400°F.
2. Transfer the potatoes cubes into a pot.
3. Add in water, makes sure they are covered.
4. Cover and bring to a boil for 2 minutes.
5. Drain any excess water.
6. Shift the potatoes to a bowl.
7. Add olive oil together with salt, black pepper, pepper, parsley and rosemary. Toss.
8. Spread them onto a baking tray in a single layer.

9. Bake until golden brown and crispy on its edges.

10. Make sure to turn over after 20 – 30 minutes.

11. Serve and enjoy.

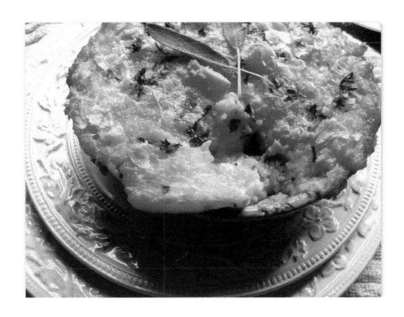

Creamy potatoes au gratin

If you like potatoes cheese, then this Mediterranean Sea diet is what you must try following the step by step method detailed below.

Ingredients

- Fresh parsley for garnish
- 5 ounces of grated cheddar
- 1 cup of heavy cream
- 2 pounds of potatoes
- 4 garlic cloves
- ½ cup of milk
- 1 teaspoon of salt
- ¼ teaspoon of black pepper

Directions

1. Preheat your oven to 400°F.
2. Place the potato slices into a large mixing dish.
3. Season with salt and pepper tossing vigorously.
4. Move it into an oven-proof dish for baking.
5. Combine cream and milk in a large jug.
6. Add crushed garlic, stir.

7. Pour this mixture over the potatoes.

8. Thoroughly move the potatoes around to coat.

9. Cover the dish with aluminum foil.

10. Let bake for 1 hour at 400°F.

11. When the timer is up, top the potatoes with grated cheese.

12. Continue to bake for another 20 minutes.

13. Let it cool briefly.

14. Serve and enjoy.

Pressure pot braised red cabbage

This recipe as a side dish goes perfectly with roasted duct, sausages and other several meals. The braising is a bit sour but healthy for consumption.

Ingredients

- 4 tablespoons of white wine vinegar
- 1 teaspoon of salt
- 3 tablespoons of granulated sugar
- 1 teaspoon of caraway seeds
- 1 small red onion
- 2 tablespoons of sunflower oil
- 1 red cabbage
- 1 cup of water

Directions

1. Start by turning on your Pressure Pot and press Sauté.
2. Add sugar and shake the inner pot to spread the sugar across the bottom equally.
3. Let the sugar melt to the point of caramelization.
4. Then, pour in the oil with onion Sauté for 1 minute.

5. Add shredded cabbage, caraway seeds, water, and salt. Stir.
6. Lock the lid and seal by the release of the valve.
7. Set the timer to 5 minutes.
8. After the 5 minutes are up, hold on for 10 minutes to release the pressure manually.
9. Now it is the right time to add the vinegar and mix.
10. Taste and adjust accordingly.
11. Serve and enjoy.

Garlic smashed potatoes

The garlic used in this recipe gives it the desired flavor and aroma. It features herbs making it most suitable for vegan.

Ingredients

- Fresh chives
- 2 pounds of baby potatoes
- ¼ cup almonds
- 1 tablespoon of salt
- 1 teaspoon of paprika
- 1 tablespoon of dried oregano
- 3 tablespoons of extra virgin olive oil
- 2 garlic cloves
- black pepper

Directions

1. Wash the potatoes and place them in a large pot.
2. Add in water and a tablespoon of salt.
3. Bring to a boil when covered.
4. Lower the heat let simmer until they are soft.
5. Heat your oven to 400°F.
6. Drain any excess water put onto a baking tray.

7. Smash the potatoes with a fork.

8. Drizzle with olive oil slightly.

9. Sprinkle each with salt and pepper.

10. Bake it on the top shelf for 20 minutes.

11. Combine 2 tablespoons of olive oil with minced garlic cloves. Mix.

12. Spread every potato with the garlic mixture.

13. Sprinkle with dried oregano, paprika, and chopped fresh chives.

14. Taste and adjust the salt accordingly.

15. Serve and enjoy as a side dish or appetizer.

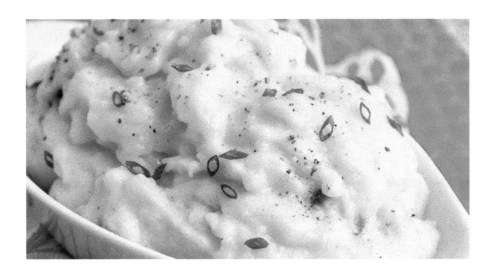

Creamy Irish colcannon

This recipe gives a new twist of smashing potatoes to creamy colcannon blended with kale and leek. It is topped with onions that also give this recipe a flavorful blast.

Ingredients

- 2 cups of packed Fresh Kale
- 2 lb. of Potatoes
- ½ cup of Milk
- 1 cup of sliced Leek
- 2 teaspoons of Salt
- ½ stick of Unsalted Butter
- A pinch of Black Pepper

Directions

1. Place prepared potatoes into a pot.
2. Add water and 2 teaspoons of salt.
3. Until they are ready.
4. As the potatoes are boiling, sauté the leek and the kale with half of the butter in a frying pan.
5. Drain any excess water after the potatoes have boiled.
6. Smash the potatoes until smooth with a fork.

7. Add in the rest of the butter together with the milk, stir well.

8. Add black pepper and salt.

9. Taste and adjust accordingly.

10. Add in the sautéed veggies and mix well.

11. If you like, top with chopped spring onions.

12. Serve and enjoy while warm.

Loaded Hassel back potatoes

These potatoes are packed with cheese and bacon with sour cream topping. They taste incredibly sweet enough to satisfy anyone's taste buds.

Ingredients

- 3 ounce of bacon strips
- 8 potatoes
- 1 tsp paprika
- 1 tablespoon of fresh parsley, chopped
- Salt and pepper
- 2 tablespoons of olive oil
- 4 ounce of cheddar cheese, sliced
- 4 tablespoons of sour cream
- 1 tsp garlic powder

Directions

1. Wash the potatoes.
2. Place 2 chopsticks on a chopping board.
3. Cut the potato severally without cutting through.
4. Move the potatoes onto a baking tray aligned with a baking paper.

5. Combine olive oil, paprika and garlic powder in a small mixing bowl.
6. Brush each potato with this mixture.
7. Season with salt and pepper.
8. Bake in an oven heated at 400°F for 55 minutes, they should be almost cooked.
9. Take the tray out.
10. Fill any existing gaps with cheese and bacon slices.
11. Put back and continue to back for 15 minutes.
12. Remove when ready, top with cheese and or fried bacon, parsley if needed.
13. Serve and enjoy.

Pear frangipane tart

Homemade pastry is a must for making pear frangipane tart from scratch with rich almond filling and tasty poached pears.

Ingredients

For pastry

- 1 egg yolk
- 1 stick unsalted butter, chilled
- 1.5 cups all-purpose flour
- 3 tablespoons of cold water
- 3 tablespoons of superfine sugar

For poached pears

- ½ cup sugar
- 3 small to medium pears
- ½ teaspoon ground cinnamon
- 2 cups water

For frangipane

- 3 medium eggs
- ⅓ cup of all-purpose flour
- 1 stick unsalted butter, diced,
- ½ cup of superfine sugar

- 1 cup of heaped ground almonds

Directions

1. In a mixing bowl, combine flour and sugar. Mix well.
2. Add butter.
3. Work the butter into the flour mixture with your hands until crumb-like texture.
4. Add egg yolk with some water.
5. Form dough with your hands.
6. Wrap and refrigerate for 1 hour.
7. As the pastry gets ready, Rinse pears and cut each in half.
8. In a small mixing dish, combine water, sugar and cinnamon.
9. Add pears mix with the mixture.
10. Bring to boil.
11. Lower the heat let simmer for 10 minutes.
12. Drain any excess water. Keep for later.
13. In another separate mixing dish, beat together butter and sugar until pale.
14. Add flour, almonds, and eggs. Mix until well combined. Set aside.
15. Divide pastry in half.
16. Roll out half of the pastry on a floured work top.
17. Transfer the pastry into oiled sandwich pan.

18. Make sure the pastry is pressed into the corners of the pan.
19. Bake in a preheated oven at 350°F for 10 minutes.
20. Remove out for filling with frangipane.
21. Top with cooked pears.
22. Transfer back in the oven.
23. Bake for 20 more minutes at the same temperature.
24. Let it cool down when ready then remove the tin.
25. Dust with powdered sugar.
26. Serve and enjoy.

Roasted white beans with vegetables the Greek style

The roasted white beans with vegetables is a true Mediterranean diet blended with garlic, tomatoes, pepper, and oregano prepared with natural olive oil.

Ingredients

- 1 tablespoon of oregano
- 1 teaspoon of tomato paste diluted with ¼ cup of water
- 1 ¼ of cup dry white beans
- Ground Pepper
- Salt to taste
- 1 red bell pepper chopped in small pieces
- 1 green bell pepper chopped in small pieces
- 1 onion grated
- 1 garlic clove slice
- ½ cup of olive oil
- 8 cherry tomatoes halved

Directions

1. Start by soaking beans a night before.

2. Clean and let beans cook by simmering for 30 minutes over medium heat.
3. Drain any excess water and keep for later.
4. Then, preheat your oven to 350 F.
5. Chop all the vegetables.
6. In a large bowl, mix the peppers together with the grated onion, oregano, garlic, beans, tomato paste mixture, olive oil, and pepper.
7. Make sure the beans to not break as you mix.
8. Add the halved cherry tomatoes, continue to mix gently.
9. Pour this mixture into a casserole dish.
10. Fill the dish with ¼ cup of hot water pouring in a corner then tilting the dish to spread the water all around.
11. Cover with aluminum foil.
12. Roast for 1 hour to soften the peppers.
13. Remove foil and continue to roast for more 10 minutes.
14. Remove, allow it to cool.
15. Add thick salt or as required.
16. Serve and enjoy with feta cheese.

Mediterranean grain bowl with lentil and chickpeas

Undoubtedly, this recipe is packed with proteins and energy giving source derived from the whole grains.

Ingredients

- 1 zucchini squash, sliced into rounds
- 3 cups of cooked faro
- 2 shallots, sliced
- 1 teaspoon of za'atar spice
- 2 avocados, skin removed, pitted and sliced
- ½ teaspoon of ground sumac
- Salt and pepper
- 1 cup of fresh chopped parsley
- Handful pitted Kalamata olives
- early harvest extra virgin olive oil
- Sprinkle crumbled feta cheese
- 2 ½ tablespoons of fresh lemon juice
- 2 cups of cooked brown lentils
- 1 garlic clove, minced
- 2 ½ teaspoons of quality Dijon mustard
- Salt

- 2 cups of cooked chickpeas
- 2 cups of cherry tomatoes, halved

Directions

1. In a non-stick pan, heat olive oil over medium-high heat until shimmering without smoke.
2. Add the sliced zucchini and Sauté on both sides to make them tender.
3. Remove the zucchini and place on a paper towel, let any excess oil drain out.
4. Season briefly with salt.
5. In a jar, add lemon juice, garlic, Dijon mustard, salt and pepper, za'atar spice, sumac, and olive oil.
6. Shale thoroughly when tightly closed. Keep for later.
7. Divide the cooked faro together with the lentils, and chickpeas equally in 4 dinner dishes.\
8. Add cooked zucchini along with the shallots, tomatoes, parsley, avocado slices, and Kalamata olives.
9. Again, season briefly with salt and pepper.
10. Drizzle with dressing on top.
11. Use the crumbled feta for finishing, if desired.
12. Serve and enjoy warm or at room temperature.

Baked lemon garlic salmon

This is an amazing recipe. The garlic fills it with its aromatic flavor.

Ingredients

- 2 teaspoons of dry oregano
- Kosher salt
- ½ teaspoon of black pepper
- ½ lemon, sliced into rounds
- 1 teaspoon of sweet paprika
- Parsley for garnish
- Zest of 1 large lemon
- 2 lb. salmon fillet
- Juice of 2 lemons
- 5 garlic cloves, chopped
- Extra virgin olive oil

Directions

1. Heat your oven to 375°F.
2. In a small mixing dish, mix together the lemon juice with garlic, lemon zest, extra virgin olive oil, paprika, oregano, and black pepper. Whisk well.

3. Organize a sheet pan. Make sure it is lined with a large piece of foil with the top brushed with extra virgin olive oil.

4. Next, pat the salmon dry, let season on both sides with kosher salt.

5. Place it on the foiled sheet pan.

6. Top with lemon garlic sauce evenly.

7. Fold foil over the salmon.

8. Then, proceed to bake for 20 minutes. The salmon should be almost cooked through on the side that is thicker.

9. Remove out and open foil to uncover the top of the salmon.

10. Place under the broiler briefly.

11. Serve and enjoy.

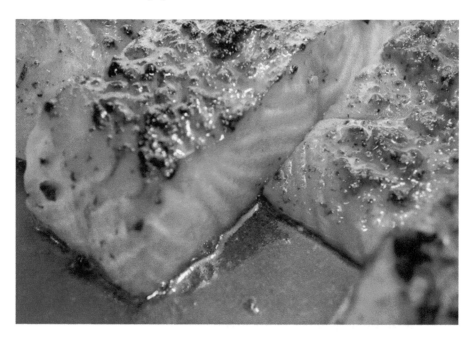

Baked fish with garlic and basil

The fish comes out tender infused with aromatic garlic flavor and the basil. It also blends in some citrus and extra virgin olive oil for a better Mediterranean diet.

Ingredients

- 2 bell peppers any color, sliced
- 15 basil leaves, sliced into ribbons
- Salt and pepper
- 1 ½ tsp dry oregano
- 2 shallots, peeled and sliced
- 1 teaspoon of ground coriander
- 10 garlic cloves, minced
- 2 lb. fish fillet
- 6 tablespoon of extra virgin olive oil
- 1 teaspoon of sweet paprika
- Juice of 1 lemon

Directions

1. Pat fish fillet dry with a kitchen towel.
2. Season with salt and pepper on every side.
3. Place the fish in a large zip-top bag.

4. Then, add the oregano, paprika, coriander, basil, minced garlic, extra virgin olive oil and lemon juice in to the bag, massage to evenly coat the fish.
5. Place in the fridge to marinated for 1 hour.
6. Heat your oven to 425°F.
7. Organize the bell peppers and shallots in the bottom of a baking dish.
8. Place the fish on top and pour the marinade over.
9. Bake in heated oven for 15 minutes.
10. Let cool briefly.
11. Serve and enjoy.

Green shakshuka recipe

This recipe is Mediterranean but takes a new classic turn with power greens especially spinach, Brussel sprouts and herbs mainly kale.

Ingredients

- Crumbled feta
- ¼ cup of extra virgin olive oil
- 1 green onion, trimmed
- 1 teaspoon of coriander
- 8 ounces of Brussels sprouts
- ½ large red onion, finely chopped
- Handful fresh parsley
- 1 teaspoon of Aleppo pepper
- 3 garlic cloves, minced
- 1 large bunch kale
- 2 cups of baby spinach
- ¾ teaspoon of cumin
- 4 large eggs
- Kosher salt
- Juice of ½ lemon

Directions

1. In a skillet that has a lid, heat the extra virgin olive oil until shimmering without smoke over medium heat.

2. Add the sliced Brussels sprouts, sprinkle with a dash of kosher salt.

3. Let cook for 6 minutes, keep tossing occasionally to soften uniformly.

4. Lower the heat.

5. Add the onions and garlic together, continue to cook for 4 more minutes, tossing regularly.

6. Add the kale, let wilt in 5 minutes as you toss.

7. Add the spinach and toss to combine.

8. Season with a pinch of kosher salt and adjust accordingly.

9. Add all the spices and toss to combine.

10. Then, add ½ cup of water.

11. Regulate the heat to medium continue to cook for 10 minutes when covered. Make sure at this point the kale is wilted totally.

12. Stir in the lemon juice.

13. Make 4 wells using your spoon.

14. Crack an egg into each well.

15. Do not forget to season each egg with some of salt. Cook for 4 minutes with the pan covered.

16. Remove from the heat.

17. Add more drizzle of extra virgin olive oil. Optional.

18. Garnish with the parsley, fresh green onions, and feta if you desire.

19. Serve and enjoy with bread or pita immediately.

Mediterranean backed cod

Unlike other recipes, the Mediterranean backed cod utilizes fewer spices mainly lemon juice, massive amount of garlic and olive oil in 15 minutes.

Ingredients

- ¾ teaspoon of salt
- ½ teaspoon of black pepper
- ¾ teaspoon of sweet Spanish paprika
- 1.5 lb. Cod fillet pieces
- ¼ cup chopped fresh parsley leaves
- 5 tablespoons of fresh lemon juice
- ¾ teaspoon of ground cumin
- 2 tablespoons of melted butter
- ⅓ cup of all-purpose flour
- 5 garlic cloves, peeled and minced
- 1 teaspoon of ground coriander
- 5 tablespoons of Private Reserve extra virgin olive oil

Directions

1. Preheat your oven ready to 400°F.

2. In a small mixing dish, mix lemon juice together with the olive oil, and melted butter. Keep for later.

3. In another separate mixing dish, mix all-purpose flour together with the spices, salt and pepper. Keep aside for later.

4. Pat fish fillet dry using a towel.

5. Dip fish in the lemon juice mixture, then dip in the flour mixture.

6. Shake off excess flour. Keep the lemon juice later.

7. In a cast iron skillet, heat 2 tablespoon of olive oil over medium temperature till shimmering without smoke.

8. Add the salmon and sear on each side. Cook briefly and remove from heat.

9. Add minced garlic to the balance of the lemon juice mixture, mix.

10. Drizzle all over the fish fillets.

11. Now you can bake in the heated oven for 10 minutes.

12. Remove from heat and sprinkle chopped parsley.

13. Serving and enjoy immediately with Lebanese rice or traditional Greek salad.

Italian oven roasted vegetables

If you are looking a massive blast of Mediterranean diet vegetables combination, then look no more. This recipe combines several vegetables that are gluten free and highly healthy.

Ingredients

- Freshly grated Parmesan cheese
- 12 ounces of baby potatoes, scrubbed
- 12 ounces of Campari tomatoes, grape
- 1 teaspoon of dried thyme
- 2 zucchini or summer squash, cut into 1-inch pieces
- 12 large garlic cloves peeled
- Extra virgin olive oil
- ½ tablespoon of dried oregano
- 8 ounces of baby Bella mushrooms cleaned, trimmed
- Salt and pepper
- Crushed red pepper flakes optional

Directions

1. Expressly, preheat your oven ready to 425°F.

2. Place the mushrooms together with the veggies and garlic in a large mixing dish.

3. Drizzle with olive oil.

4. Add the thyme, dried oregano, salt, and pepper. Toss to combine.

5. Only take the potatoes and spread them on a baking pan slightly oiled.

6. Roast for 10 minutes in the preheated oven.

7. Add the mushrooms together with the remaining vegetables after removing the potatoes from the oven.

8. Return to the oven for further 20 minutes roasting or until the veggies are tender.

9. If you desire, sprinkle with of freshly grated Parmesan cheese.

10. Serve and enjoy immediately.

Shrimp pasta recipe
Mediterranean diet style

Shrimp pasta is flavored with garlic, onions, and lemon juice. It gets ready in only 20 minutes.

Ingredients

- 1 lemon zested and juiced
- Kosher salt
- 1 lb. of large shrimp peeled and deveined
- Parmesan cheese to your liking
- ½ red onion chopped
- ¾ lb. of thin spaghetti
- 1 teaspoon of dry oregano
- 3 vine ripe tomatoes chopped
- Black pepper
- ½ teaspoon of red pepper flakes
- Extra virgin olive oil
- 1 cup of dry white wine
- 5 garlic cloves minced
- Large handful chopped fresh parsley

Directions

1. Begin by cooking the pasta in salted boiling water as per the manufacturers instruction on the package.
2. Drain any excess water and reserving some for later.
3. As the pasta is cooking, in a large pan heat extra virgin olive oil over medium temperature until it shimmers without smoke.
4. Cook the shrimp for 3 minutes on each side until pink.
5. Shift the shrimp to a side plate.
6. In the same pan, reduce the heat to medium-low.
7. Then, add the onions together with the oregano, garlic, and red pepper flakes.
8. Continue to cook for further 2 minutes, stirring constantly.
9. Add the wine to the pan, be sure to scrape up any pieces of garlic and onions.
10. Cook the wine briefly.

Stir in the lemon juice and lemon zest.

11. Add the chopped parsley and tomatoes, toss vigorously for 15 seconds.
12. Season with Kosher salt and adjust accordingly.
13. Now, add the cooked pasta to the pan, let toss to coat.
14. Then, add some of the reserved pasta starchy water.
15. Add the cooked shrimp.
16. Allow the shrimp to warm through briefly.

17. Remove from heat and sprinkle a little grated parmesan cheese and red pepper flakes.
18. Serve and enjoy immediately.

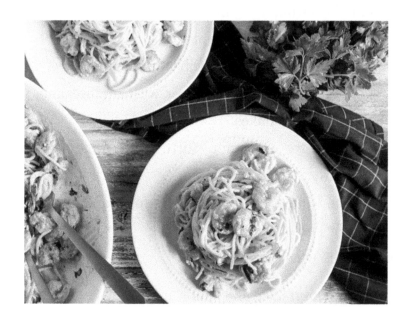

Moroccan vegetable tagine recipe

In this recipe, the Moroccan flavors take control of the taste with vegetables stew packed balance. The recipe is gluten free with vegetables and fruits.

Ingredients

- 10 garlic cloves, peeled and chopped
- 2 large russet potatoes, peeled and cubed
- 1 lemon, juice of
- 1 large sweet potato, peeled and cubed
- 1 teaspoon of ground cinnamon
- Handful fresh parsley leaves
- Salt
- 1 teaspoon of ground coriander
- ¼ cup of Private Reserve extra virgin olive oil
- 2 medium yellow onions, peeled and chopped
- 1 tablespoon of Harissa spice blend
- ½ teaspoon of ground turmeric
- 2 cups of canned whole peeled tomatoes
- 2 large carrots, peeled and chopped
- ½ cup of heaping chopped dried apricot

- 1 quart of low sodium vegetable broth
- 2 cups cooked chickpeas

Directions

1. Heat oil over low heat until just shimmering without smoke in a large pot.
2. Add onions and increase heat to medium.
3. Then, Sauté for 5 minutes, tossing frequently.
4. Now add the garlic and the chopped veggies.
5. Season with salt and spices. Toss again to combine.
6. Cook this combination for 7 minutes on medium-high temperature, regularly stir with a wooden spoon.
7. Add tomatoes together with the apricot and broth.
8. Season again with small dash of salt.
9. Maintain the heat on medium-high, continue to cook for 10 more minutes.
10. Then lower the heat to simmer when covered for 25 minutes or until veggies are tender.
11. Next, stir in chickpeas let cook for 5 minutes more on low heat.
12. Stir in lemon juice and fresh parsley.
13. Taste and adjust accordingly.
14. Shift to serving dishes topping each with a drizzle of Private Reserve extra virgin olive oil.
15. Serve and enjoy with couscous or rice.

Easy homemade spaghetti sauce

This is purely a vegetarian spaghetti sauce and can be made ahead of time.

Ingredients

- Bit of dried oregano
- Torn basil and chopped fresh parsley
- 1 medium sized onion
- pinch of sweet paprika
- 4 garlic cloves, minced.
- 2 carrots
- Extra virgin olive oil
- A large 28-ounce can of crushed tomatoes

Directions

1. In a pot, add 2 tablespoons of extra virgin olive oil.
2. Heat over medium temperature until shimmering without smoke.
3. Add chopped onions together with the garlic and finely grated carrots.
4. Cook for 5 minutes while stirring frequently.

5. Add in crushed tomatoes to the mixture with some bit of water.
6. Season with kosher salt and black pepper accordingly.
7. Stir in dry oregano together with the paprika, basil, and parsley.
8. Bring to a boil briefly, then reduce heat.
9. Cover with a lid to simmer for 20 minutes.
10. To let the pasta, absorb some flavors, cover and leave for 6 minutes.
11. Serve and enjoy.

Loaded Hassel back potatoes

These potatoes are packed with cheese and bacon with sour cream topping. They taste incredibly sweet enough to satisfy anyone's taste buds.

Ingredients

- 3 ounce of bacon strips
- 8 potatoes
- 1 tsp paprika
- 1 tablespoon of fresh parsley, chopped
- Salt and pepper
- 2 tablespoons of olive oil
- 4 ounce of cheddar cheese, sliced
- 4 tablespoons of sour cream
- 1 tsp garlic powder

Directions

1. Wash the potatoes.
2. Place 2 chopsticks on a chopping board.
3. Cut the potato severally without cutting through.
4. Move the potatoes onto a baking tray aligned with a baking paper.

5. Combine olive oil, paprika and garlic powder in a small mixing bowl.

6. Brush each potato with this mixture.

7. Season with salt and pepper.

8. Bake in an oven heated at 400°F for 55 minutes, they should be almost cooked.

9. Take the tray out.

10. Fill any existing gaps with cheese and bacon slices.

11. Put back and continue to back for 15 minutes.

12. Remove when ready, top with cheese and or fried bacon, parsley if needed.

13. Serve and enjoy.

Fig tart

Figs fruits are the essential ingredients in making this recipe. It blends puff pastry and ricotta along with fig filling. This recipe is perfect for a Mediterranean desert in about 25 minutes.

Ingredients

- 1 puff of pastry sheet, thawed
- 8 ounces of ricotta
- 3 tablespoons of honey
- 12 fresh figs
- 4 tablespoons of almonds , roughly chopped
- 2 teaspoons of shredded coconut

Directions

1. Preheat your oven to 400°F.
2. Mix ricotta together with the honey and figs flesh until well combine in a small dish. Keep for later.
3. Unfold the pastry and roll it out thin.
4. Cut in half.
5. Place all of them onto a baking tray aligned with baking parchment.
6. Cut indentations alongside the edges.

7. Between the two tarts, divide the ricotta mixture and spread over. Make sure the mixture is only in the inner frame cut with the knife.

8. Then cut 2 figs into wedges.

9. Put them on the tart randomly.

10. Then, put the tray in the oven.

11. At 400°F, bake for 12 minutes, the edges should become puffed and the bottom should turn golden brown.

12. Cut each fig into 8 pieces.

13. The almonds should be roughly chopped.

14. Take the tarts out when they are ready.

15. Use the fresh figs for topping, then sprinkle with almonds and coconut.

16. Serve and enjoy warm.

Pear frangipane tart

Homemade pastry is a must for making pear frangipane tart from scratch with rich almond filling and tasty poached pears.

Ingredients

For pastry

- 1 egg yolk
- 1 stick unsalted butter, chilled
- 1.5 cups all-purpose flour
- 3 tablespoons of cold water
- 3 tablespoons of superfine sugar

For poached pears

- ½ cup sugar
- 3 small to medium pears
- ½ teaspoon ground cinnamon
- 2 cups water

For frangipane

- 3 medium eggs
- ⅓ cup of all-purpose flour
- 1 stick unsalted butter, diced,
- ½ cup of superfine sugar

- 1 cup of heaped ground almonds

Directions

1. In a mixing bowl, combine flour and sugar. Mix well.
2. Add butter.
3. Work the butter into the flour mixture with your hands until crumb-like texture.
4. Add egg yolk with some water.
5. Form dough with your hands.
6. Wrap and refrigerate for 1 hour.
7. As the pastry gets ready, Rinse pears and cut each in half.
8. In a small mixing dish, combine water, sugar and cinnamon.
9. Add pears mix with the mixture.
10. Bring to boil.
11. Lower the heat let simmer for 10 minutes.
12. Drain any excess water. Keep for later.
13. In another separate mixing dish, beat together butter and sugar until pale.
14. Add flour, almonds, and eggs. Mix until well combined. Set aside.
15. Divide pastry in half.
16. Roll out half of the pastry on a floured work top.
17. Transfer the pastry into oiled sandwich pan.

18. Make sure the pastry is pressed into the corners of the pan.

19. Bake in a preheated oven at 350°F for 10 minutes.

20. Remove out for filling with frangipane.

21. Top with cooked pears.

22. Transfer back in the oven.

23. Bake for 20 more minutes at the same temperature.

24. Let it cool down when ready then remove the tin.

25. Dust with powdered sugar.

26. Serve and enjoy.

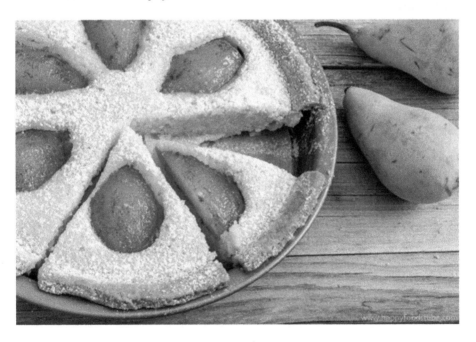

Roasted white beans with vegetables the Greek style

The roasted white beans with vegetables is a true Mediterranean diet blended with garlic, tomatoes, pepper, and oregano prepared with natural olive oil.

Ingredients

- 1 tablespoon of oregano
- 1 teaspoon of tomato paste diluted with ¼ cup of water
- 1 ¼ of cup dry white beans
- Ground Pepper
- Salt to taste
- 1 red bell pepper chopped in small pieces
- 1 green bell pepper chopped in small pieces
- 1 onion grated
- 1 garlic clove slice
- ½ cup of olive oil
- 8 cherry tomatoes halved

Directions

1. Start by soaking beans a night before.
2. Clean and let beans cook by simmering for 30 minutes over medium heat.
3. Drain any excess water and keep for later.
4. Then, preheat your oven to 350 F.
5. Chop all the vegetables.
6. In a large bowl, mix the peppers together with the grated onion, oregano, garlic, beans, tomato paste mixture, olive oil, and pepper.
7. Make sure the beans to not break as you mix.
8. Add the halved cherry tomatoes, continue to mix gently.
9. Pour this mixture into a casserole dish.
10. Fill the dish with ¼ cup of hot water pouring in a corner then tilting the dish to spread the water all around.
11. Cover with aluminum foil.
12. Roast for 1 hour to soften the peppers.
13. Remove foil and continue to roast for more 10 minutes.
14. Remove, allow it to cool.
15. Add thick salt or as required.
16. Serve and enjoy with feta cheese.

Mediterranean grain bowl with lentil and chickpeas

Undoubtedly, this recipe is packed with proteins and energy giving source derived from the whole grains.

Ingredients

- 1 zucchini squash, sliced into rounds
- 3 cups of cooked faro
- 2 shallots, sliced
- 1 teaspoon of za'atar spice
- 2 avocados, skin removed, pitted and sliced
- ½ teaspoon of ground sumac
- Salt and pepper
- 1 cup of fresh chopped parsley
- Handful pitted Kalamata olives
- early harvest extra virgin olive oil
- Sprinkle crumbled feta cheese
- 2 ½ tablespoons of fresh lemon juice
- 2 cups of cooked brown lentils
- 1 garlic clove, minced
- 2 ½ teaspoons of quality Dijon mustard
- Salt

- 2 cups of cooked chickpeas
- 2 cups of cherry tomatoes, halved

Directions

1. In a non-stick pan, heat olive oil over medium-high heat until shimmering without smoke.
2. Add the sliced zucchini and sauté on both sides to make them tender.
3. Remove the zucchini and place on a paper towel, let any excess oil drain.
4. Season briefly with salt.
5. In a jar, add lemon juice, garlic, Dijon mustard, salt and pepper, za'atar spice, sumac, and olive oil.
6. Shale thoroughly when tightly closed. Keep for later.
7. Divide the cooked faro together with the lentils, and chickpeas equally in 4 dinner dishes.\
8. Add cooked zucchini along with the shallots, tomatoes, parsley, avocado slices, and Kalamata olives.
9. Again, season briefly with salt and pepper.
10. Drizzle with dressing on top.
11. Use the crumbled feta for finishing, if desired.
12. Serve and enjoy warm or at room temperature.

Lebanese rice with vermicelli

Ingredients

- ½ cup toasted pine nuts, to finish, though optional
- Water
- 2 cups of long grain
- 1 cup broken vermicelli pasta
- Salt
- 2 ½ tablespoon of olive oil

Directions

1. Ultimately, start by rinsing the rice properly.
2. Put the rinsed rice in a medium bowl and cover with water let soak for 15 – 20 minutes.
3. Make sure you are able to easily break the grain of rice with your thumbs, drain all the water.
4. Heat the olive oil on medium temperature in a medium non-stick cooking pot.
5. Add the vermicelli and continuously stir to equally toast it.
6. Make sure the vermicelli should transform to a golden brown color with intensive supervision to prevent burning.

7. Add the rice and continue to stir so that the rice will be well-coated with the olive oil.

8. Season with salt.

9. Add 3 ½ cups of water and bring it to a boil until the water reduces in size.

10. Reduce the heat significantly low and keep the rice covered.

11. Continue to cook for 15 – 20 minutes on that low heat.

12. When the rice is completely cooked switch off the heat

13. Simmer the rice for 10 – 15 minutes in its pot.

14. Uncover and fluff with a fork

15. Serve and top with toasted pine nuts.

16. Enjoy.

Greek style baked cod with lemon and garlic

In only 15 minutes you would have finished to bake this Greek style cod with lemon and garlic with handful of spices and much garlic to give it an attractive aroma and taste.

Ingredients

- ½ teaspoon of black pepper
- ¾ teaspoon of sweet Spanish paprika
- 1.5 lb. Cod fillet pieces about 4 or 6 pieces
- 5 tablespoons of fresh lemon juice
- 5 peeled and minced garlic cloves
- 1 teaspoon of ground coriander
- ¾ teaspoon of ground cumin
- 2 tablespoons of melted butter
- ¼ cup chopped fresh parsley leaves
- 5 tablespoons of Private Reserve extra virgin olive oil
- ⅓ cup all-purpose flour
- ¾ teaspoon of salt

Directions

1. Preheat oven to 400°F.

2. After, mix the lemon juice with olive oil, and melted butter in a shallow bowl.

3. Keep aside, safely.

4. In a separate second shallow bowl, mix all-purpose flour, salt, spices, and pepper, then also set a side just next to the lemon juice mixture.

5. Pat fish the fillet dry.

6. To coat, dip fish in the lemon juice mixture, and also dip in the flour mixture.

7. Endeavor to shake off any excess flour.

8. Keep the remaining lemon juice mixture for later.

9. In a cast iron skillet, heat 2 teaspoon of olive oil over medium-high temperature to until shimmering without smoke.

10. Add fish and sear on both side to give color. Cook for few minutes on every side.

11. Take off the heat.

12. Add minced garlic to the remaining lemon juice mixture and blend.

13. Then drizzle all over the fish fillets.

14. Bake in the heated oven for 10 minutes or until it begins to flake easily when tapped with a fork.

15. Take off the heat and sprinkle with chopped parsley.

16. Serve immediately preferable with Lebanese rice, traditional Greek salad or any other salad of your choice.

17. Enjoy.

One pan Mediterranean baked halibut with vegetables recipe

This exact halibut is made simply with green beans and cherry tomatoes in only 25 minutes.

Citrus, fresh garlic and other spices give it a flavorful delicious taste to shake one's taste buds.

Ingredients

- ½ - ¾ teaspoon of ground coriander
- Zest of 2 lemons
- 1 teaspoon of seasoned salt, more for later
- 1 lb. cherry tomatoes
- 1 ½ lb. halibut fillet, sliced into about 1 ½-inch pieces
- 1 ½ tablespoon of freshly minced garlic
- ½ teaspoon of ground black pepper
- 1 cup Private Reserve Greek extra virgin olive oil
- 1 teaspoon of dried oregano
- 1 lb. fresh green beans
- 2 teaspoon of dill weed
- Juice of 2 lemons
- 1 large yellow onion sliced into half moons

Directions

1. Preheat your oven to 425°F.
2. Begin by whisking the sauce ingredients together, in a large mixing bowl.
3. Add the green tomatoes, beans, and onions toss to coat with the whisked sauce
4. Using a large slotted spoon, move the vegetables to a large baking sheet
5. Keep the vegetables to one side of the baking sheet. Spread out in only one layer.
6. You can proceed to add the halibut fillet strips to the remaining sauce then toss to enabling coating.
7. Move the halibut fillet to the baking sheet right next to the vegetables.
8. Pour any remaining sauce on top.
9. Lightly sprinkle the halibut and vegetables with seasoned salt.
10. Start to bake in the already heated oven for 15 minutes.
11. Move the baking sheet to the top oven rack
12. Broil for more 3 minutes with close supervision to prevent burning until when the cherry tomatoes pop right under the broiler.
13. Remove the baked halibut and vegetables from the oven when ready
14. Serve and enjoy.

Moroccan fish recipe

An equivalent of braised cod recipe, the Moroccan fish recipe is a game changer in regards to sweetness and deliciousness of this recipe.

Made in thick tomato sauce, chickpea and pepper with several other healthy Moroccan Mediterranean flavors, you do not want to miss out on this recipe; try out for yourself.

Ingredients

- 1 ½ lb. cod fillet pieces
- 1 ½ cup water
- Extra Virgin Olive Oil
- ½ teaspoon of cumin
- 2 tablespoon of tomato paste
- ½ lemon juice
- ½ lemon, sliced into thin rounds
- 2 medium tomatoes, diced
- 1 red pepper, cored, sliced
- ¾ teaspoon of paprika
- 1 15-oz. can chickpeas, drained and rinsed
- Kosher salt and black pepper
- Large handful fresh cilantro
- 8 garlic cloves, divided minced and sliced 4 for each

- 1 ½ teaspoon of Ras El Hanout , should be divided

Directions

1. In a large pan with cover, start by heating 2 tablespoons of extra virgin olive oil over medium temperature until shimmering without smoke.
2. Add minced garlic let cook shortly of course while tossing frequently until fragrant.
3. Add diced tomato, tomato paste, and bell peppers continue to cook for 3 – 4 minutes in a medium temperature and again keep tossing frequently.
4. Add water, cilantro, chickpeas, and sliced garlic let season with kosher salt and pepper.
5. Stir in ½ teaspoon of Ras El Hanout spice mixture.
6. Increase the heat and boil.
7. Bring down the heat and cover part-way an let simmer for 20 minutes. It is absolutely okay to add water if necessary.
8. Whereas, combine the remaining cumin with Ras El Hanout , paprika in a small bowl.
9. Season the fish with kosher salt and pepper and the spice mixture on either sides.
10. Add a drizzle of the extra virgin olive oil.
11. Check to see that all the fish is properly coated with the spices and the olive oil.

12. Add the season fish to the pan, when ready, then nestle the fish pieces into the saucy chickpea and tomato mixture.
13. Add lemon juice and lemon slices.
14. Cook content for more 10 – 15 minutes on a low temperature until content is completely cooked.
15. Garnish with fresh cilantro.
16. Serve as soon as possible with crusty bread or rice.

Baked chicken recipe

No doubt chicken is one of the world's favorite dishes that is deliciously enjoyed by millions to billions of people.

The baked chicken uses spicy garlic and fresh basil as well as parsley to keep you hanging on the dish forever.

Ingredients

- 1 medium red onion, halved and thinly sliced
- 44.4 ml Extra virgin olive oil
- 5 – 6 Campari tomatoes halved
- Fresh basil leaves for garnish
- Juice of ½ lemon
- Salt and pepper
- 3.6 g dry oregano
- 1 teaspoon of fresh thyme
- 907.185g of boneless skinless chicken breast
- 2.1g Sweet paprika
- 4 garlic cloves, minced
- Handful chopped fresh parsley for garnish

Directions

1. Begin by preheating your oven to 425°.
2. Firstly, pat the chicken dry.

3. Put the chicken breast in a large zip-top then zip it after releasing air that might be in bag.
4. Put it on a poultry chopping board, pound with meat mallet until the chicken flattens.
5. Remove out of the zip-top bag, repeat the process with all the remaining chicken breast pieces.
6. Season chicken with salt and pepper on every side, then put in a large mixing bowl.
7. Add spices, extra virgin olive oil, minced garlic, and lemon juice.
8. Combine to ensure the chicken is equally coated with the spices and garlic.
9. Oil a large baking dish very lightly, then spread onion slices on the bottom.
10. Organize seasoned chicken on top after which add the tomatoes to it.
11. Tightly cover the baking dish with a foil let bake for 10 minutes.
12. Then uncover, continue to bake for more 8 – 10 minutes. Nevertheless, this step may take more that the specified time according to the thickness of your chicken breast.
13. Take off the source of heat.
14. Keep covered with a pan for more 5 – 10 minutes before you serve
15. Uncover and garnish with fresh parsley and basil.
16. Serve and enjoy

Mediterranean shrimp recipe

The shrimp is perfectly coated in Mediterranean spices with skillet cooked in a tasty white wine olive oil sauce that contains shallots, tomatoes and peppers.

This should take less than 25 minutes and its ready for you bite.

Ingredients

- 1 ¼ lb. large shrimp peeled and deveined
- 1 tablespoon of butter
- 3 tablespoons of Private Reserve extra virgin olive oil
- 1 Lebanese Rice recipe
- ½ teaspoon of ground coriander
- 2 tablespoons of dry white wine
- ½ teaspoon of each salt and pepper
- 4 garlic cloves, chopped
- ½ green bell pepper
- 2 teaspoons of smoked Spanish paprika
- ⅓ cup chopped parsley leaves
- 1 tablespoon of all-purpose flour
- ¼ teaspoon of cayenne
- 1 cup canned diced tomato
- ⅓ cup chicken or vegetable broth
- ¼ teaspoon of sugar

- 3 shallots thinly sliced
- ½ yellow bell pepper sliced
- 2 tablespoons of fresh lemon juice

Directions

1. Start by preparing the Lebanese rice as per the package
2. Keep covered and undisturbed until ready to serve.
3. Pat shrimp dry then put it in a large bowl.
4. Add flour, salt, smoked paprika, pepper, cayenne, coriander, and sugar.
5. Toss until shrimp is fully coated on all sides.
6. In a large heavy frying pan, heat to melt the butter together with the olive oil over medium temperature.
7. Introduce the shallots and garlic to the content let cook for 2 – 3 minutes as you stir till fragrant.
8. Add bell peppers continue to cook for more 4 minutes while tossing infrequently.
9. Place the shrimp in the content and cook for 1 – 2 minutes.
10. Add the diced broth, tomatoes, white wine and lemon juice.
11. Let cook for 5 minutes till when the shrimp turns bright orange.
12. Stir in chopped fresh parsley.
13. Serve soon enough with the cooked rice you started with.

14. Enjoy.

Baked lemon garlic salmon recipe

Ingredients

- Zest of 1 large lemon
- Extra virgin olive oil
- Kosher salt
- Parsley for garnish
- 5 garlic cloves, chopped
- 2 teaspoon of dry oregano
- ½ lemon, sliced into rounds
- 1 teaspoon of sweet paprika
- 2 lb. salmon fillet
- 3 tablespoon of extra virgin olive oil
- Juice of 2 lemons
- ½ teaspoon of black pepper

Directions

1. Begin by heating your oven to 375 °.
2. Secondly, make the lemon-garlic sauce.

3. In a small bowl, mix together the lemon zest, lemon juice, oregano, extra virgin olive oil, garlic, paprika and black pepper.

4. Whisk the sauce to perfection.

5. Organize your sheet pan lined with a large piece of foil that can fold over to cover the salmon.

6. Brush top of the foil with extra virgin olive oil.

7. Pat salmon dry, then season properly on all sides with kosher salt.

8. Put it on the foiled sheet pan.

9. Top with the already made lemon garlic sauce.

10. Fold foil over the salmon covering the whole salmon.

11. Let bake for 15 – 20 minutes until salmon is about to be cooked through at the thickest part. Nonetheless, the 15 – 20 minutes is directly dependent on the thickness of the salmon.

12. Be vigilant to ensure that it is not over cooked.

13. Gently, remove from oven, open foil to uncover the top of the salmon.

14. Briefly put salmon under the broiler for 3 minutes.

15. Make sure the garlic does not burn due to over broiling.

16. Serve and enjoy.

Sheet pan chicken and vegetables

This chicken is a perfect combination with vegetables and no fuss but tossed with oregano, citrus, and of course garlic that masterminds the flavor and unique taste. This vegetable chicken is a beautifully sweet and healthy option for Mediterranean diet lovers.

Ingredients

- Extra virgin olive oil
- 1 large red pepper, cored and cut to chunks
- 1 teaspoon of Paprika
- 1 lemon, zested and juiced
- 2 teaspoon of dry oregano
- 1 teaspoon of white vinegar
- 1 red onion, cut into chunks
- 9 baby broccoli, trimmed and cut into equal pieces
- 1 ½ lb. boneless chicken breast
- 1 teaspoon of coriander
- 5 garlic cloves, minced
- Kosher salt and black pepper

- 2 medium zucchini halved length-wise, sliced into crescent shape of a moon
- Fresh parsley for garnish, optional

Directions

1. Heat your oven to about 400°.
2. Put all the cut vegetables in a large mixing bowl.
3. Then add chicken pieces together with the minced garlic.
4. Season with kosher salt and black pepper.
5. Add spices.
6. Add lemon juice, lemon zest, vinegar, drizzle generously with extra virgin olive oil.
7. Toss properly to ensure perfect combining. Furthermore, endeavor to ensure that the vegetables and chicken pieces are equally coated.
8. Move content to a large sheet pan and spread well in only one layer.
9. Begin baking in the ready heated oven for 20 minutes or until the chicken is totally cooked through.
10. You can garnish with fresh parsley before you continue to serve.
11. Enjoy.

Sicilian style fish stew recipe

This Mediterranean diet dish is packed with Italian flavors to heighten its delicacy. It is best in white wine-tomato broth, capers and garlic among other ingredients.

Ingredients

- Salt
- Pepper
- ¾ cup of dry white wine
- 4 large garlic cloves, minced
- ½ teaspoon dried thyme
- 2 lb. skinless sea bass fillet cut into large cubes
- Crusty Italian bread for serving
- ¼ cup of golden raisins
- Pinch red pepper flakes
- 1 large yellow onion, chopped
- 2 tablespoon of rinsed capers
- ½ cup chopped fresh parsley leaves
- 2 celery ribs, chopped
- 3 cups of low-sodium vegetable broth
- Extra virgin olive oil
- 1 28-oz. can of whole peeled plum tomatoes, juice separated and reserved

- 3 tablespoons of toasted pine nuts, optional

Directions

1. Start by heating 1 tablespoon of olive oil in 5-quart oven over medium temperature.
2. Add celery, onions, and a small salt and pepper.
3. Cook while regularly stirring until softened in for 4 minutes.
4. Add thyme, red pepper flakes and garlic continue to cook shortly until fragrant enough only in 30.
5. Stir in the white wine and reserved tomato juice from a can.
6. Simmer briefly then continue cooking until the liquid reduces significantly by ½.
7. Add the vegetable broth, tomatoes, raisins, and capers.
8. Cook for more 15 – 20 minutes on a medium temperature until flavors are fully combined.
9. Pat the fish dry, then proceed to season lightly with the salt and pepper.
10. Carefully fix pieces of fish into the already cooking liquid then stir gently to nicely cover the fish pieces in the cooking liquid.
11. Simmer for some time, continue to cook for more 5 minutes.
12. Remove content from source of heat and cover.

13. Let settle off heat for more 4 – 5 minutes to ensure swift cooking of all the pieces of fish.

14. Make sure the fish is flaky enough when gently pulled apart from the sauce with a knife or fork.

15. Lastly, you can stir in the chopped parsley.

16. Pour the hot fish stew into serving bowls immediately to top with toasted pine nuts if desired.

17. Serve with crusty bread

18. Enjoy.

Greek chicken souvlaki with tzatziki

Believe me not, this recipe will remind you of the last time you had it for dinner in streets of Athens. You most likely would want to make your own because you are now far away from their yet the taste of this amazing recipe keeps calling your name. below are the ingredients and complete step-by-step Directions.

Ingredients

- 2 bay leaves
- Greek pita bread
- Sliced tomato
- 1 teaspoon of each Kosher salt and black pepper
- Tzatziki Sauce
- ¼ cup dry white wine
- Juice of 1 lemon
- 2 ½ lb.. of organic boneless skinless chicken breast, no fats and cut into 1 ½ inch pieces
- 2 tablespoons of dried oregano
- 10 garlic cloves, peeled
- sliced cucumber
- 1 teaspoon of dried rosemary

- ¼ cup of Greek extra virgin olive oil
- sliced onions
- Kalamata olives
- 1 teaspoon of sweet paprika

Directions

1. Begin by preparing the marinade.
2. In a small food processor bowl, add oregano, pepper, garlic, paprika, rosemary, salt, white wine, olive oil, and lemon juice, then pulse thoroughly to combine.
3. Add bay leaves to chicken put in a separate large bowl.
4. Top it with marinade toss thoroughly to ensure that it is fully combined.
5. Ensure chicken is properly and evenly coated.
6. Cover tightly and refrigerate for 2 hours
7. Get 10 – 12 wooden skewers, then soak properly in water for 30 – 45 minutes.
8. Proceed to prepare the tzatziki sauce including all other fixings.
9. Thread marinated chicken pieces through the prepared skewers when the tzatziki sauce is ready.
10. Organize the outdoor grill
11. Brush with a small oil and heat over medium temperature.

12. Put the chicken skewers on grill until well browned, keeping regulating inside temperature around 155° on the monitoring thermometer for 5 minutes.
13. Keeping brushing with marinade, discard any leftovers.
14. Move the chicken to serving area let cool for 3 minutes.
15. Warm the pitas through.
16. Arrange chicken souvlaki pitas after spreading with tzatziki sauce on the pita, add chicken pieces and lastly add the vegetables and olives.
17. Enjoy.

Grilled swordfish with a Mediterranean twist

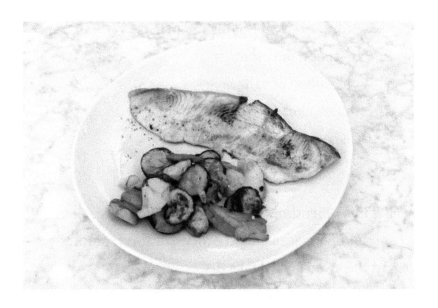

The swordfish recipe highly relies on the delicious marinade of the Mediterranean pumped with fresh garlic cloves, cumin among others flavorful ingredients.

Try to make this at home with the following ingredients and step-by-step directions below.

Ingredients

- 4 swordfish steaks

- ¾ teaspoon of cumin
- ½ tsp freshly ground black pepper
- ⅓ cup extra virgin olive oil
- 6 to 12 garlic cloves, peeled
- ½ to 1 tsp sweet Spanish paprika
- 1 teaspoon of coriander
- ¾ teaspoon of salt
- 2 tablespoon of fresh lemon juice
- Crushed red pepper, optional

Directions

1. Begin by blending the olive oil, garlic, spices, lemon juice, salt and pepper in a food processor for 3 minutes.
2. Pat the swordfish steaks dry
3. Place the dry swordfish steaks in a pan to generously apply the marinade on every side after which keep aside for 15 minutes as the grill heats up
4. Oil the grates and preheat a gas grill with high temperature.
5. When properly heat, grill the fish steaks on high temperature for 5 – 6 minutes on one side and so the other side until the fish can easily flake when tapped with a fork.
6. Use a splash of lemon juice to finish and sprinkle with crushed red pepper flakes as desired.
7. Serve and enjoy.

Greek shrimp recipe with tomato and feta

The flavors in this recipe are fully packed. It includes fresh herbs, tomato sauce, feta as well as olive. This dish is served with crusty bread or even favorite grains.

Ingredients

- 1 ½ teaspoon of dry dill weed, divided
- Pinch red pepper flakes
- 2 56g crumbled Greek feta cheese
- 6 garlic cloves, minced, divided
- 1 ½ teaspoon of dry oregano, divided
- Chopped fresh mint leaves
- Greek extra virgin olive oil
- Juice of ½ lemon
- Black pepper
- 6 pitted Kalamata olives, optional
- 1 large red onion, chopped
- 1 ½ lb. large shrimp fully thawed, peeled and deveined
- Kosher salt
- 1 737.088g canned diced tomato, drain only some of the liquid

- Chopped fresh parsley leaves

Directions

1. Pat shrimp dry, put in a large bowl.
2. Season with kosher pepper, salt, ½ teaspoon of dry oregano, pinch red pepper flakes, ½ teaspoon of dry dill weed, and ½ teaspoon of minced garlic.
3. Drizzle with the extra virgin olive oil
4. Toss thoroughly to fully combine keep aside.
5. In a large skillet, heat 2 teaspoon of extra virgin olive oil on medium heat until shimmering without smoke.
6. Add chopped onion together with all the remaining minced garlic then cook shortly while stirring frequently until fragrant.
7. Add tomatoes together with the lemon juice
8. Season with a pinch of pepper, salt, dill, and the remaining dry oregano.
9. Boil
10. Reduce the heat to medium to allow simmering for 15 minutes.
11. Introduce the marinated shrimp.
12. Continue to cook for 5 – 7 minutes
13. Now it is time to stir in fresh mint and parsley leaves.
14. Sprinkle the feta and black olives to finish.
15. If desired, add a splash of lemon juice according to your taste preference.
16. Serve over plain orzo or your favorite crusty bread.

Mediterranean sautéed shrimp and zucchini

Ingredients

- 1 teaspoon of ground coriander
- 1 lb. large shrimp
- ½ teaspoon of sweet paprika
- Kosher salt
- 1 ½ cups cherry tomatoes, halved
- Handful fresh basil leaves, torn or sliced into ribbons
- ½ medium red onion, thinly sliced
- 5 garlic cloves, minced and divided
- Extra virgin olive oil
- 2 zucchini halved and sliced into ½ moons
- 1 teaspoon of ground cumin
- 1 ½ tablespoon of dry oregano
- Pepper
- 1 cup cooked chickpeas drained
- 1 bell pepper, cored and sliced into sticks
- 1 large lemon juice

Directions

1. Combine cumin, coriander, oregano, and paprika in a small bowl.
2. Pat shrimp dry and season with 1 ½ tsp of the spice mixture and kosher salt.
3. Set aside in a refrigerator mainly if you will use at a later time. Ensure to keep some spice mixture for the veggies.
4. Heat 2 tablespoon of extra virgin olive oil over medium temperature in a large cast iron skillet.
5. Add½ the amount of garlic together with the onions let cook for 3 – 4 minutes keep tossing regularly until fragrant.
6. Add the bell peppers, zucchini, and chickpeas together for seasoning with pepper and salt together with the remaining spice mixture.
7. Toss to combine and blend.
8. Increase the heat if deemed necessary continue to cook the veggies until tender of course keep tossing regularly for 5 – 7 minutes.
9. Move all the vegetable to large plate for the moment.
10. Take back the skillet to the heat, add small extra virgin olive oil.
11. Add the seasoned shrimp and remaining garlic.
12. Cook over medium temperature while stirring occasionally in 4 – 5 minutes till shrimp is totally pink

13. Return the cooked vegetables back to the skillet that contains the shrimp.

14. Add cherry tomatoes and lemon juice.

15. Toss once again and finish with fresh basil.

16. Serve and enjoy.

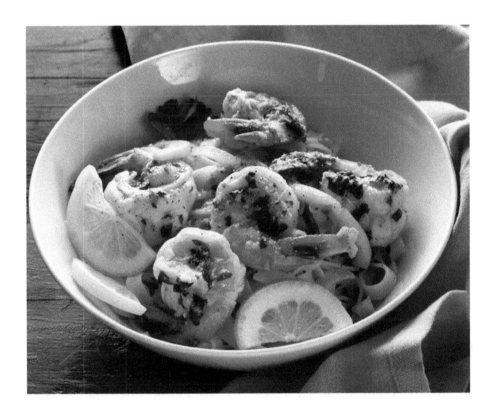

Mediterranean salmon kabobs

Ingredients

- 1 teaspoon of ground cumin
- 3 minced garlic cloves
- 1 zucchini, sliced into rounds
- 1 small red onion, cut into squares
- Kosher salt and pepper
- ½ teaspoon of ground coriander
- 1.5 lb. Salmon fillet, cut into cubes
- 1 lemon, zested, juiced
- 2 teaspoons of chopped fresh thyme leaves
- ¼ - ⅓ cup of extra virgin olive oil
- 2 teaspoons of dry oregano
- 1 teaspoon of mild chili pepper

Directions

1. In a small bowl, begin by whisking together all the marinade ingredients of extra virgin olive oil, thyme, oregano, Aleppo pepper, lemon juice and zest, garlic, cumin, and coriander.
2. In a large mixing bowl, put the salmon pieces, onions, and zucchini for seasoning with kosher salt and pepper. Do not forget to toss briefly.

3. Carefully pour the marinade over the salmon and toss again to ensure total coating of the with the marinade.

4. Leave to marinate for 15 – 20 minutes

5. Thread the salmon and other ingredients typically onions and zucchini by the use of skewers.

6. Arrange and heat the outdoor grill

7. Arrange salmon skewers on top and cover the grill.

8. Grill salmon kabobs for 6 – 8 minutes keep covered till fish is completely opaque. Endeavor to turn over halfway when cooking.

9. Serve when hot or at room temperature.

10. Enjoy.

Greek chicken and potatoes

This recipe is quite best for a family with hidden secrets in the lemon garlic sauce. Marinade the chicken for some hours or alternatively you can prepare it directly without marinade, the taste will remain remarkably sweeter.

Ingredients

- 1 teaspoon of black pepper
- ¼ cup of extra virgin olive oil
- Salt
- ½ teaspoon of ground nutmeg
- 4 gold potatoes clean, cut into thin wedges
- 6 – 12 pitted quality Kalamata olive oil
- Fresh parsley, for garnish
- 1 lemon, sliced
- ¼ cup of lemon juice
- 1 cup of chicken broth
- 12 fresh garlic cloves, minced
- 1 medium yellow onion, halved and sliced
- 3 lb. of chicken pieces, bone in with the skin
- 1 ½ tablespoon of dried rosemary

Directions

1. Preheat your oven ready to 350°.
2. Pat chicken dry and season with salt
3. Organize the potato wedges and onions in the bottom of a baking dish.
4. Season with 1 teaspoon of black pepper and salt.
5. Add the chicken pieces to the seasoned potato wedges.
6. Make the lemon-garlic sauce.
7. Whisk ¼ cup extra virgin olive oil with lemon juice together with minced garlic, rosemary, and nutmeg in a small bowl.
8. Pour all over the chicken and potatoes evenly.
9. Organize lemon slices on top.
10. Pour chicken broth into the pan from one side. However, be mindful not to pour the broth on the chicken.
11. Transfer to the preheated oven while uncovered for 45 minutes - 1 hour until tender at 165°.
12. Add Kalamata together with olives when removed from heat source.
13. You can garnish with some bit of fresh parsley accordingly.
14. Serve and enjoy salads and tzatziki sauce.

Mediterranean baked fish recipe with tomatoes and capers

Ingredients

- ⅓ cup of golden raisins
- ⅓ cup of Greek extra virgin olive oil
- 2 large tomatoes, diced
- Fresh parsley or mint for garnish
- 10 garlic cloves, chopped
- Juice of ½ lemon
- 1 ½ teaspoon of organic ground coriander
- Zest of 1 lemon
- 1 teaspoon of all-natural sweet Spanish paprika
- ½ tsp cayenne pepper
- 1 ½ tablespoon of capers
- Salt and pepper
- 1 small red onion, chopped
- 1 teaspoon of organic ground cumin
- 1 ½ lb. of white fish fillet

Directions

1. Begin right away by preparing the tomato and capers sauce.

2. Heat extra virgin olive oil on medium temperature to shimmer without smoke in a medium saucepan.
3. Add onions let cook for 3 minutes until turns golden in color of course tossing regularly.
4. Add garlic, pinch of salt, spices, tomatoes, capers, pepper, and raisins.
5. Bring to a boil
6. Lower the heat down to medium-low allow it to simmer for 15 minutes.
7. Heat your oven to 400°.
8. Pat fish dry and season with salt and pepper on every sides.
9. Pour ½ of the cooked tomato sauce into the bottom of a baking dish.
10. Arrange the fish on top.
11. Add lemon juice and lemon zest.
12. Top with all the remaining tomato sauce.
13. Bake in the heated oven for 15 – 18 minutes.
14. Remove from then garnish with fresh parsley or mint accordingly
15. Serve hot with zucchini, Lebanese rice or potatoes.

Roasted beet hummus

Roasted beet hummus is perfect protein rich dip. It is roasted in an oven yet nutritious and it takes 40 minutes to get ready.

Ingredients

- 2 tablespoon of tahini
- 1½ lemon, juice only
- Salt to taste
- 2 cups of cooked chickpeas
- 1 garlic clove
- 3 fresh beets
- 4 tablespoon of olive oil
- ¼ cup water

Directions

1. Clean and cut the beets into chunks.
2. Put them on a baking tray.
3. Drizzle with bit of olive oil.
4. Then bake in a preheated oven at 400°F for not less than 40 minutes.
5. Let cool.

6. Mix all remaining ingredients in a food processor together with the cooled beets.
7. Process until smooth.
8. Serve and enjoy with a dip.

Vegetarian fresh spring rolls with peanut sauce

This particular Mediterranean recipe is fully packed with vegetables both raw and cooked perfect for a vegan lover. It is highly refreshing.

Ingredients

- 1 small lemon
- 2 tablespoons of honey
- 2 medium carrots
- 2 tablespoons of water
- 2 cups of baby kale leaves
- ¼ head of purple cabbage
- 1 teaspoon of soy sauce
- 4 tablespoons of peanut butter
- 6 rice paper sheets
- 1 large red bell pepper
- 2 medium avocados
- Feta cheese

Directions

1. Place warm water in a large frying pan.

2. Place in a cup of rice to soak until it becomes soft in approximately 30 seconds.

3. Add the fillings down on the soft paper placed on a clean work top.

4. Crumble feta cheese over.

5. Next bit of peppers, carrots, and cabbage.

6. Roll the fillings in the paper the same way you would make a wrap.

7. Nevertheless, roll enough to close the first batch of fillings.

8. When the filling has reduced make more with avocado and cabbage to properly stuff the rolls.

9. Place the fillings on your hands and at the same time roll the roll away from you while tucking the fillings in.

10. To close the edges, simply fold the wrapper in.

11. Combine peanut butter, lemon, honey, soy sauce and water. Blend until smooth.

12. Serve and enjoy immediately.

Warm Buddha bowl

Warm Buddha features lentil, broccoli, avocado, lettuce and tomatoes. These ingredients make a perfect Mediterranean diet.

Ingredients

- 5 tablespoons of extra virgin olive oil
- 1 tablespoons of olive oil
- 2 cups of lamb lettuce
- 1 cup of cherry tomatoes
- A pinch of salt
- ½ cup of water
- 2 cups of broccoli florets
- 1 cup of cooked lentils
- 1 cup of fresh spinach
- 2 teaspoons of butter
- A pinch of salt
- 1 tablespoons of sweet paprika
- 2 teaspoon of black sesame seeds
- 1 ripe large avocado
- 6 sun-dried tomatoes, soaked in water

Directions

1. Place oil in a large frying pan.
2. Add cherry tomatoes together with broccoli florets, let roast for 3 minutes.
3. Gather them to one side of the pan.
4. Add butter together with the salt and paprika mix.
5. Let cook for extra 3 minutes then switch off the heat.
6. Cut your avocado into slices.
7. Fill your bowls with avocado and lettuce.
8. Add roasted veggies and lentils topping with the sesame seeds.
9. Combine spinach, sundried tomatoes, virgin oil, salt, and water in a food processor and pulse until smooth for dressing.
10. Serve and enjoy.

Tomato salsa shrimp and rice

Rice is a perfect Mediterranean recipe for dinner. It is a quick and juicy meal.

Ingredients

- 3 tablespoon of extra virgin olive oil
- 1 cup of rice
- Salt to taste
- ½ onion
- 1 garlic cloves
- ½ cup of fresh flat leaf parsley
- 5 ripe tomatoes
- 1 cup of fresh shrimp
- 2 tablespoon of unsalted butter

Directions

1. Prepare your rice normally or as instructed on the package.
2. Add parsley, tomatoes, garlic, onion, and oil in a food processor.
3. Blend or process until very smooth.
4. In a pan, melt butter place in the shrimp.
5. Cook for 2 minutes, then add salsa continue to boil.

6. Lower the heat and simmer until when the mixture becomes slightly thick.
7. Taste and adjust accordingly.
8. Serve and enjoy.

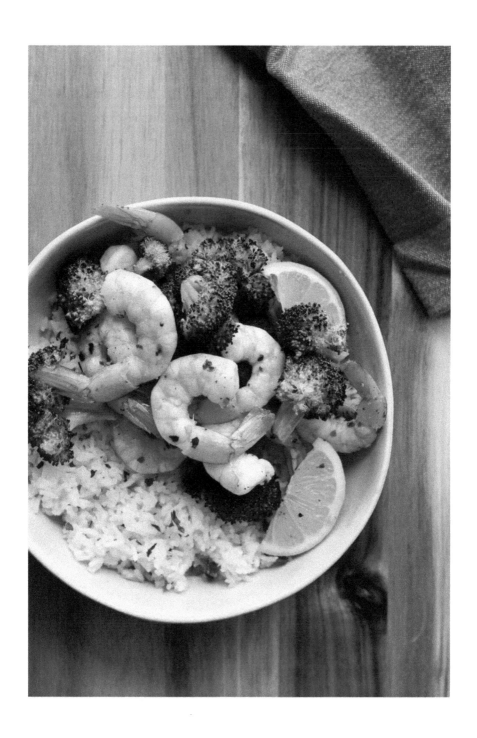

Lightning Source UK Ltd.
Milton Keynes UK
UKHW020841040621
384920UK00001B/103